Homemade Beauty Products
Easy DIY Recipes & Holistic Solutions
for
Glowing Skin and Beautiful Hair

By Cassia Albinson

Disclaimer:

A physician has not written the information in this book. Although natural therapies are generally safe to use, if you suffer from any serious medical condition, are pregnant, or on medication you should consult your doctor first to see if you can apply it. This book is for informational and educational purposes only.

All information in this book has been carefully researched and checked for factual accuracy. However, the author and publishers make no warranty, expressed or implied, that the information contained herein is appropriate for every individual, situation or purpose, and assume no responsibility for errors or omission. The reader assumes the risk and full responsibility for all actions, and the author will not be held liable for any loss or damage, whether consequential, incidental, and special or otherwise that may result from the information presented in this publication.

If you are pregnant or have any serious health condition, do not use any aromatherapy treatments described in this book without consulting with your physician and aromatherapy practitioner first.

TABLE OF CONTENTS

Home Made Beauty Products: Introduction 1

Chapter One Homemade Moisturizers 8

AROMATHERAPY & ESSENTIAL OILS PRECAUTIONS 9

Aromatherapy General Precautions 9

Orange Essential Oil Moisturizer 11

Juniper Berry Essential Oil Moisturizer 12

Melissa Essential Oil Moisturizer 13

Lavender Essential Oil Moisturizer 14

Sage Essential Oil Moisturizer 15

Eucalyptus Essential Oil Moisturizer 16

Lemongrass Essential Oil and Honey Moisturizer 17

Chapter Two Homemade Facial Masks 19

Avocado and Banana Facial Mask 20

Coconut Oil Facial Mask with Orange Essential Oil 22

.... 23

Honey, Ginger and Coconut Oil Facial Mask 24

Avocado, Honey and Burdock Root Facial Mask 26

Pomegranate Juice and Olive Oil Facial Mask 28

Coconut Oil and Melissa Essential Oil Facial Mask 30

Chapter Three Homemade Body Scrubs 32

Epsom Salt and Orange Essential Oil Body Scrub 33

.... 34

Epsom Salt and Eucalyptus Essential Oil Body Scrub 35

Epsom Salt and Juniper Berry Essential Oil Body Scrub 37

Organic Sea Salt and Coconut Oil Body Scrub 38

.... 39

Organic Sea Salt and Olive Oil Body Scrub 40

Organic Sea Salt and Avocado Oil Body Scrub 41

Organic Sea Salt, Ginger and Lemongrass Essential Oil Body Scrub.. 43

Organic Sea Salt and Melissa Essential Oil Body Scrub............ 45

Chapter Four Homemade Hair Care Products............................. 46

Coconut Oil Hair Treatment 47

.... 48

Coconut Oil and Orange Essential Oil Hair Treatment............. 49

Apple Cider Vinegar Volumizing Hair Treatment...................... 51

Olive Oil and Lavender Essential Oil Hair Treatment 53

Conclusion 55

Home Made Beauty Products: Introduction

The commercial cosmetic industry is one of the largest and wealthiest industries in the world and it provides us with products to suit all different skin types, cosmetic needs and wants. There are many benefits to these products that range from ant-aging properties; skin nourishing properties; hair nourishing properties; moisturizing properties; cleansing properties and toning properties. All of these properties and benefits provided by products that are manufactured by the commercial cosmetic industry have become a necessity to our daily lives and beauty routines; not only because we are all searching for that magic elixir that will ensure us eternal youth, but also because the environmental factors of the world we live in today are unavoidable and many of these factors can cause harm to our skin. We therefore need to make sure that we take care of our skin and hair in as many ways as we possibly can.

Unfortunately beauty products that are provided by the commercial cosmetic industry have many draw backs. The first of these draw backs is their cost; many of these products, although they are of top quality, can be very expensive and therefore cost-prohibitive for many of us. Another of these draw backs is that commercially produced cosmetics are generally chemically derived and therefore contain a list of ingredients that most of us can't even pronounce let alone know what they are. Then there is the fact that so many of these commercially produced cosmetics are high in synthetic fragrances that are added to the products in order to mask the harsh and unpleasant fragrance of the chemicals from which they are derived. These chemicals and synthetic fragrances can cause serious irritation to sensitive skins and have been known to cause irritation and sensitivity to skin types that are not normally prone to such reactions.

One of the most important and sensitive issues surrounding the production of commercial cosmetic products is the fact that many of the huge worldwide cosmetic corporations are known to test their products on live animals in order to make sure that they are aware of any potential reactions that the consumer may have to the use of a particular product. This is a very sore point the world over and many women are beginning to seek alternative options when it comes to beauty products and cosmetics as they do not want to in any way promote such cruel and unnecessary practices.

The good news is that there is an alternative option to the cosmetics and beauty products that are produced by the commercial industry, and therefore a means of avoiding all their previously mentioned draw backs. It is very easy, cost-effective and rewarding to make your own beauty products within the comfort of your own home and by doing so not only are you taking complete control of exactly what you are putting onto your skin and into your hair, but you are also providing your skin and hair with naturally derived ingredients that won't cause harm or irritation.

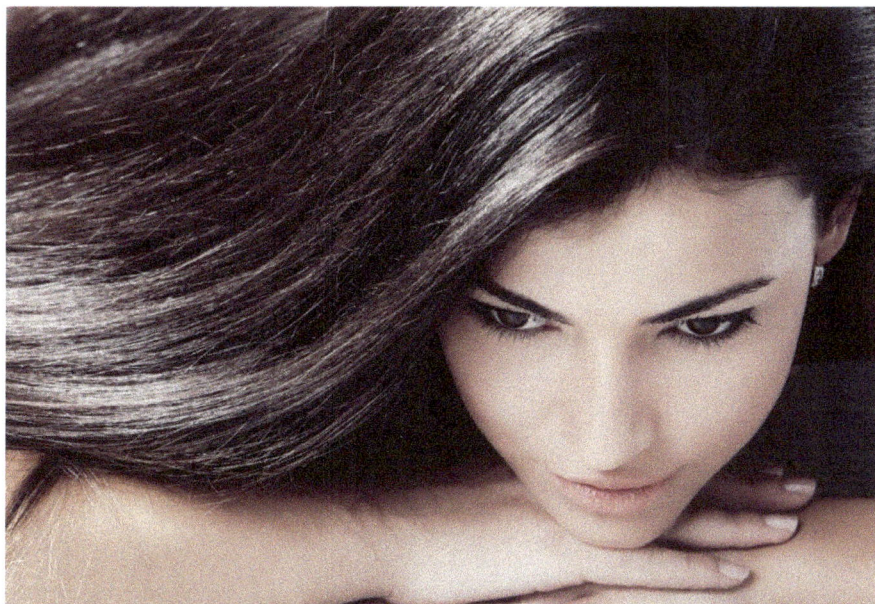

The aim of this book is to provide you with cost-effective, natural and creative alternatives to the everyday commercially produced cosmetics that we are so used to using, but don't necessarily have to. The recipes for homemade beauty products in this book will provide you with a number of options for moisturizing, cleansing and exfoliating your skin; as well as a number of options for moisturizing, cleansing and treating your hair. All the ingredients in these recipes are naturally sourced with the exception of the moisturizers which use plain, basic aqueous cream as a base; however some would argue that aqueous cream is derived from natural products, especially when it is in its most basic and clean form.

As far as fragrances are concerned, the recipes in this book use essential oils as a means of adding fragrance to the products; this not only takes away the risk of causing irritation to the skin that would be done by the use of synthetic fragrance, but it also adds to the products all the benefits that come with the use of the essential oils.

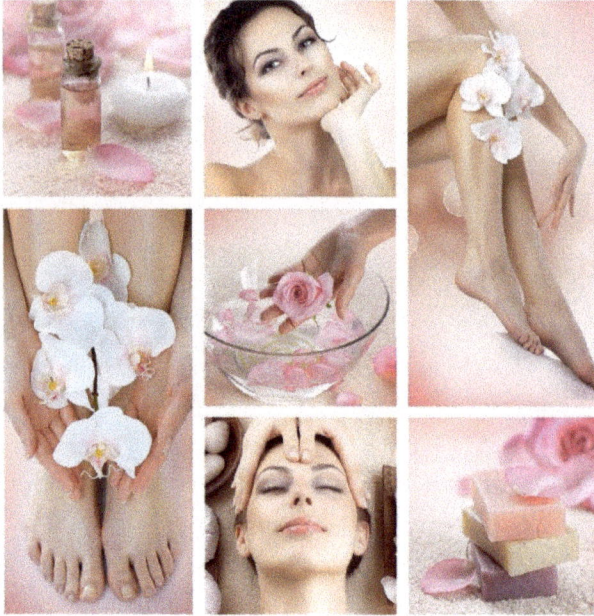

Some of the products in this book will need to be made and used immediately, particularly in the case of some of the face masks; otherwise many of them can be stored in airtight glass jars and used when, and as often, as desired.

The following chapters of will provide you with creative, cost-effective and easy to make recipes for moisturizers, face masks, body scrubs, hair treatments as well as cleansing products for both skin and hair.

It is important to note that although all the ingredients in the recipes to follow are natural and non-chemical, it is still known that some skin types may have allergic reactions to some of the ingredients so it is always important to perform a sensitivity test before using the homemade product. To perform this sensitivity test, place a small amount of the completely made-up product on the inside of your forearm and allow it to sit there for approximately twenty minutes before washing off. Even if an allergic reaction does not occur immediately there is still a chance that it can develop, therefore it is advised that you wait at least twenty four hours before using the product again in order to completely ensure that you will not develop any potential allergic reactions or sensitivities to the product or its ingredients.

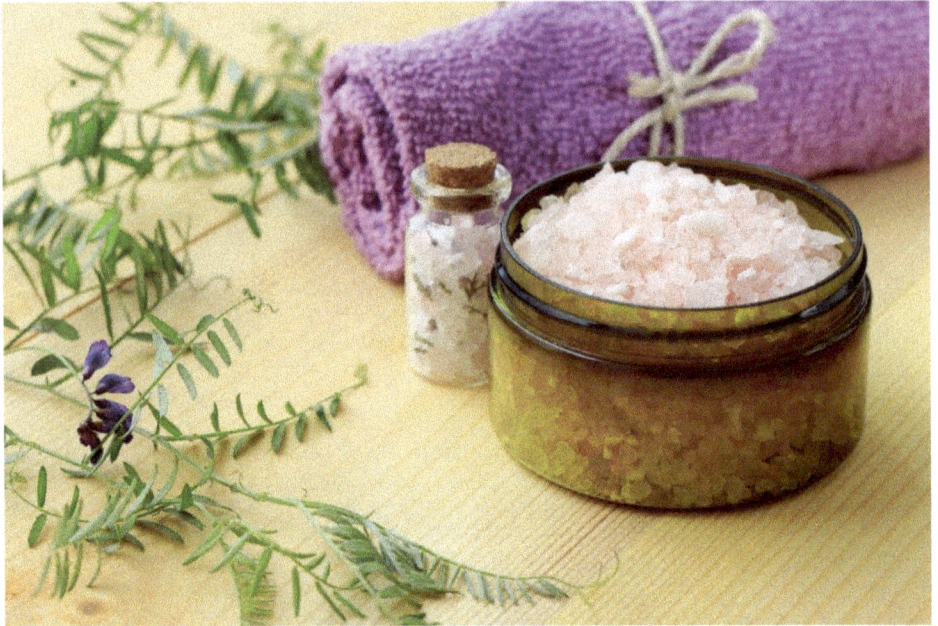

It is also important to note that if you are already aware that you may have, or do have, a sensitivity to any of the ingredients in the recipes that follow then it would be advisable to avoid the use of the recipe completely.

In the event of an allergic reaction or sensitivity occurring to any of the products within the recipes that does not clear up or heal within at least three days of use, then it is strongly advised that you consult with your doctor or dermatologist regarding the reaction and completely discontinue use of the homemade product.

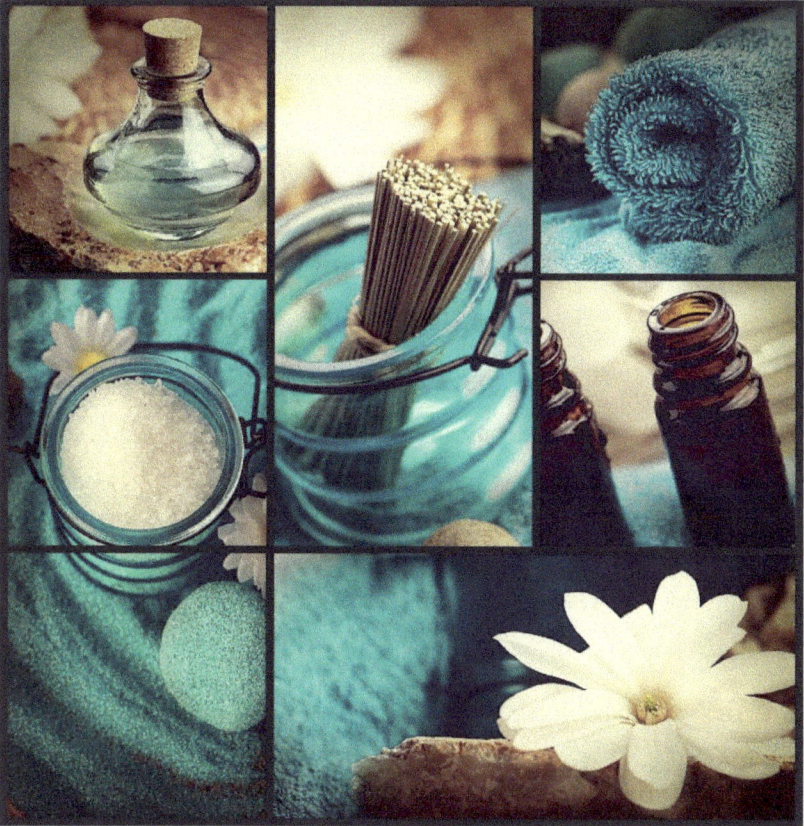

Chapter One
Homemade Moisturizers

The recipes for homemade moisturizers in this section can be used for both face and body and all of them use plain, basic aqueous cream as their base. Aqueous cream is known for its gentle yet effective moisturizing properties and abilities and is one the most basic options for effectively moisturizing the skin since it has a neutral pH level that is not likely to cause any reaction or sensitivity to the skin. The addition of essential oils to these recipes adds a hint of fragrance as well as the benefits of the particular essential oil that is being used in each circumstance. All of these recipes can be put together and stored in an airtight container, preferably recycled glass, and used as and when needed. They can also be placed in smaller containers that are easy to keep in your handbag, since they make great hand moisturizers as well. Once again it is important to remind you of the precautions mentioned in the introduction regarding potential allergic reactions or sensitivities to any of these recipes. Should any reactions or sensitivities occur discontinue use immediately.

AROMATHERAPY & ESSENTIAL OILS PRECAUTIONS

Aromatherapy General Precautions

Aromatherapy is a very safe and easy therapy to use, but keep in mind that there are certain precautions:

- Remember to wash your hands after applying aromatherapy massage;

- Do not apply the essential oils in their pure form as they may cause an allergic reaction. Instead, use blends that contain 2-5% essential oils diluted in good-quality cold-pressed oil;

-After using citrus oils, like for example lemon, verbena, bergamot, orange etc. avoid direct sun exposure, even up to 8 hours after the treatment

- Do not apply oils after surgery (unless you have consulted with a doctor) or on open wounds or rashes of unknown origin;

- Do not use the oils after chemotherapy (unless suggested by a doctor);

- Keep the oils away from the eyes and mucus membranes;

- Use the oils only topically (unless you have consulted with an aromatherapist who specializes in phytoaromatherapy);

- Avoid rosemary, thyme, Spanish and common sage, fennel and hyssop if you suffer from high blood pressure;

- Do not apply the treatments described in this book on babies or infants. It doesn't mean that aromatherapy can never be used on babies and infants, but extremely low concentrations should be used. Always consult with a medical or naturopathy doctor first;

- After an aromatherapy massage always remember to wash your hands;

- Make sure that you research the brand, read safety instructions for each individual oil you buy/use and check the expiration date;

- Store your blends in dark glass bottles, preferably in a cool, dry and dark place and remember to use within a maximum of one month after mixing.

Orange Essential Oil Moisturizer

Orange essential oil has many health benefiting properties such as anti-inflammatory, anti-depressant, anti-spasmodic, it is a natural antiseptic, a carminative, can have a sedative-like effect, can be used as a diuretic, and a general health tonic. Orange essential oil is also known for its anti-ageing properties. The citrus fragrance of the orange essential oil is believed to promote a calm state as well as that of creativity, making this a great fragrance to add to a moisturizer that you will be using at the beginning of the day.

Ingredients:

- 2 Cups (500ml) Plain aqueous cream

- 2 Tablespoons (30ml) Orange essential oil

Instructions:

1. In a mixing bowl that you have set aside for using with non-food products, place the plain aqueous cream

2. Add the orange essential oil and mix well.

3. Place the mixture into a recycled glass jar and use as and when desired for both face and body, preferably after cleansing the skin.

Juniper Berry Essential Oil Moisturizer

Juniper berry essential oil is known for its health benefiting properties such as; it is an antiseptic, anti-rheumatic, antispasmodic, calmative, and a diuretic. With its anti-rheumatic properties juniper berry oil will be a great addition to aqueous cream to make a moisturizing mixture that will help relieve aching, tired joints and muscles making this moisturizer combination a great way to round off your after-training shower or bath. Juniper Berry Essential oil has a woody fragrance that is known and believed to promote a calm state of mind.

Ingredients:

- 2 Cups (500ml) Plain aqueous cream

- 2 Tablespoons (30ml) Juniper Berry essential oil

Instructions:

1. In a mixing bowl that you have set aside for using with non-food products, place the plain aqueous cream

2. Add the Juniper Berry essential oil and mix well.

3. Place the mixture into a recycled glass jar and use as and when desired for the body. Due to the anti-rheumatic properties of the juniper berry oil, this moisturizer is a wonderful remedy to stiff, tired muscles so it will make a great rub for the releasing of muscles after intense exercise and when used in this instance it will be most effective after a hot bath.

Melissa Essential Oil Moisturizer

Melissa essential oil is known for its health benefiting properties such as; it is an antidepressant, has sedative-like properties, is a calmative and has hyposensitive properties. The hyposensitive properties of the Melissa essential oil make it a great addition to any moisturizer that is intended for use on sensitive skin, or skin that is prone to allergic reactions.

Ingredients:

- 2 Cups (500ml) Plain aqueous cream

- 2 Tablespoons (30ml) Melissa essential oil

Instructions:

1. In a mixing bowl that you have set aside for using with non-food products, place the plain aqueous cream

2. Add the Melissa essential oil and mix well.

3. Place the mixture into a recycled glass jar and use as and when desired for the body, preferably after a bath or shower.

Lavender Essential Oil Moisturizer

Lavender essential oil is known for its health benefiting properties such as its ability to relieve and eliminate nervous tension, relieve pain, disinfect the skin and enhance respiratory function. The addition of lavender essential oil to this moisturizer makes it a great way to end off a long hot bath while you are attempting to recover from an illness such as the common cold or influenza.

Ingredients:

- 2 Cups (500ml) Plain aqueous cream

- 2 Tablespoons (30ml) Lavender essential oil

Instructions:

1. In a mixing bowl that you have set aside for using with non-food products, place the plain aqueous cream

2. Add the Lavender essential oil and mix well.

3. Place the mixture into a recycled glass jar and use as and when desired for the body, preferably after a bath or shower.

Sage Essential Oil Moisturizer

Sage essential oil is known for its health benefiting properties such as; it is an antifungal, antimicrobial, anti-oxidant, antiseptic, antibacterial and anti-inflammatory. Due to its natural cleansing properties that won't be harsh and irritating to the skin, the addition of sage essential oil to this moisturizer makes it a great handbag essential for use as a hand cream. This is a very useful hand and body moisturizer for active and sportspeople as it will help ensure that you are cleansing your skin of any bacteria that is caused by sweating, without stripping the skin of its natural oils or being too abrasive. When using this moisturizer after a bath or shower you are further ensuring that your skin is well cleansed without any concern of having been to abrasive in the process.

Ingredients:

- 2 Cups (500ml) Plain aqueous cream

- 2 Tablespoons (30ml) Sage essential oil

Instructions:

1. In a mixing bowl that you have set aside for using with non-food products, place the plain aqueous cream

2. Add the Sage essential oil and mix well.

3. Place the mixture into a recycled glass jar and use as and when desired for the body, preferably after a bath or shower.

Eucalyptus Essential Oil Moisturizer

Eucalyptus essential oil is known for its health benefits that include; anti-inflammatory, antispasmodic, antiseptic, and antibacterial. When combined with the high magnesium content of the Epsom salt, eucalyptus essential oil makes a great addition to any moisturizer or body care product that will be used by active people and sportspeople. This moisturizer also uses pure aqueous cream as a base, so it won't cause any irritation to sensitive skin.

Ingredients:

- 2 cups (500ml) Pure aqueous cream

- 2 Cups (500ml) Epsom Salt

- ¼ Cup (60ml) Eucalyptus Essential Oil

Instructions:

1. Using a glass jar or a recycled aqueous cream tub, place the aqueous cream into the jar or tub

2. Add the Epsom salt

3. Add the eucalyptus essential oil

4. Mix together well

5. Use as desired on hands and body, preferably after cleansing

Lemongrass Essential Oil and Honey Moisturizer

Lemongrass essential oil is known for its health benefiting properties such as; it is an analgesic, antidepressant, antimicrobial, antiseptic, astringent, antibacterial and antifungal. Lemongrass essential oil is also known as a calmative, diuretic, insect repellent and has deodorizing properties. Honey is one of nature's best antibacterial ingredients and is known to help boost the immune system as well. Honey is also known for its own moisturizing properties as well as its antiseptic properties. With all these benefits, lemongrass essential oil makes a great ingredient for any homemade moisturizer, and together with all the benefits of the honey, this moisturizer is useful to all walks of life. With its natural cleansing and antibacterial, as well as its insect repelling properties, this homemade moisturizer will be great to use all over your body and perfect for keeping in your handbag so that you have some with you all the time. The combination of the fragrances between the lemongrass essential oil and the honey gives this moisturizer a very comforting appeal to the olfactory senses.

Ingredients:

- 2 Cups (500ml) Plain aqueous cream

- 2 Tablespoons (30ml) Lemongrass essential oil

- 2 Tablespoons (30ml) Raw organic honey

Instructions:

1. In a mixing bowl that you have set aside for using with non-food products, place the plain aqueous cream

2. Add the Lemongrass essential oil and the honey, and mix well.

3. Place the mixture into a recycled glass jar and use as and when desired for the body, preferably after a bath or shower.

Chapter Two
Homemade Facial Masks

The homemade facial masks in this chapter are all made with natural food-based products that not only have benefits for the body from within, but can also benefit the body from without. Since most of these recipes use fresh food sources it is recommended that you use these masks as you make them; however when it comes to the necessity of performing a sensitivity test on your skin it is possible to make these masks and then keep them in the refrigerator for the required twenty four hours that it will take to fully complete the sensitivity test. When storing these masks in the refrigerator it is recommended that you store them in an airtight container such as a recycled glass jar. As with all the recipes and chapters in this book it is important and necessary to once again stress the fact that if any irritation or sensitivity occurs through use of the products that these recipes make, use of the product must be discontinued immediately; further more if there is any reaction to the product or any of its ingredients that does not clear up within three days of the initial reaction, it is strongly advised that you consult your doctor or dermatologist.

Avocado and Banana Facial Mask

Avocados are known for their high vitamin E content and therefore are an incredibly effective natural moisturizer for the skin. Bananas, as with avocados, are high in potassium and antioxidants both of which promote the regeneration and repair of muscle fiber and tissues. This mask is a wonderful option when you are looking to both hydrate your skin and fight the signs of aging as the moisturizing benefits from the avocado in conjunction with the high potassium levels of both ingredients will work as one to help plump up the skin and reduce fine lines and wrinkles that are caused by skin dehydration.

Ingredients:

- 1 Small ripe avocado, pitted and peeled

- 1 Small ripe banana, peeled

Instructions:

1. Place the avocado and banana into a mixing bowl

2. Mash the avocado and banana together to form a smooth paste

3. Cleanse your face by means of your usual cleansing routine

4. Apply the avocado and banana facial mask to your face and neck, extending all the way down to your décolletage.

5. Leave the mask on until it begins to dry and harden

6. Gently remove the mask by wiping away at it with a dampened cotton wool pad

7. Follow with your usual cleansing and moisturizing routine.

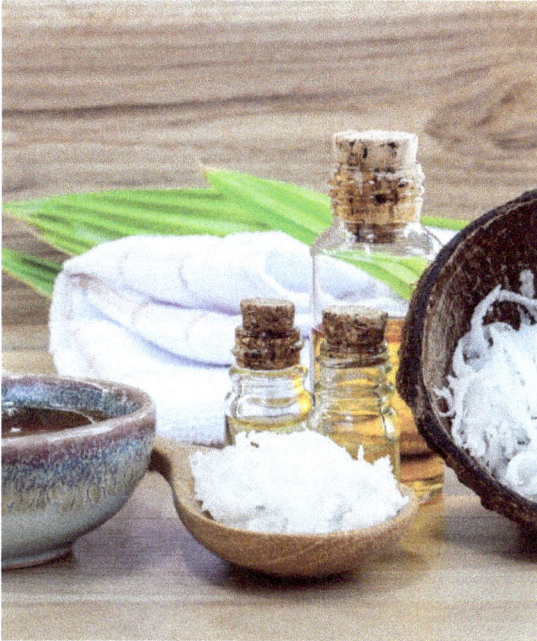

Coconut Oil Facial Mask with Orange Essential Oil

Coconut oil is another of those super food ingredients that has benefits for the body from both within and without. Since coconut oil is high in healthy unsaturated fats it makes for an incredibly efficient and cost-effective skin moisturizer that doesn't leave the skin feeling oily and unclean. Orange essential oil is known for its anti-aging properties and is high in anti-oxidants, making this combination an incredibly good source of age-defying natural ingredients.

Ingredients:

- 1 Tablespoon (15ml) Extra virgin coconut oil, preferably in its more solid state

- ½ teaspoon (2.5ml) Orange essential oil

Instructions:

1. Place the coconut oil and the orange essential oil in a mixing bowl and mix together well

2. Cleanse your face and neck by means of your usual cleansing routine

3. Apply the coconut oil and orange essential oil facial mask to your face and neck, extending down to your décolletage.

4. Leave the mask on for approximately fifteen minutes

5. Gently remove the mask by wiping away at it with a dampened
   cotton wool pad

6. Follow with your usual cleansing and moisturizing routine.

Honey, Ginger and Coconut Oil Facial Mask

Honey is another of those super food ingredients that has been used for medicinal purposes for centuries, particularly within the Chinese culture, and it is renowned and celebrated for its anti-bacterial and anti-inflammatory properties. The naturally occurring ingredient found in honey called populous is known for its cleansing properties which are the reason why honey is an ingredient in so many cleansing products. Ginger is well known for its anti-inflammatory and anti-bacterial properties as well. The combination of honey and ginger provides a good dose of age fighting anti-oxidants to this facial mask. By using coconut oil as a base for this recipe you are providing your skin with a moisturizing mask that is both anti-aging and deep cleansing at the same time, making this facial mask a wonderful addition to any make-up removing beauty routine.

Ingredients:

- 1 Tablespoon (15ml) Extra virgin coconut oil, preferably in its solid state

- 1 teaspoon (5ml) Raw organic honey

- ½ teaspoon (2.5ml) Fresh ginger root, finely grated

Instructions:

1. Place the coconut oil, honey and ginger into a mixing bowl and mix well

2. Cleanse your face and neck by means of your usual cleansing routine

3. Apply the honey, ginger and coconut oil facial mask to your face and neck, extending down to your décolletage.

4. Leave the mask on for approximately fifteen minutes

5. Gently remove the mask by wiping away at it with a dampened cotton wool pad

6. Follow with your usual cleansing and moisturizing routine.

Avocado, Honey and Burdock Root Facial Mask

Burdock root has been traditionally used in the ancient art of healing known as Ayurvedic Medicine, which is a medicinal system that is native to India and the sub-content. Ayurvedic practice uses burdock root to treat skin conditions such as rashes, acne, abscesses, local skin infections, eczema and psoriasis. The Ayurvedic philosophy believes burdock root to be one of nature's greatest skin cleansers. The combination of burdock root and honey in this facial mask make it a wonderful homemade, non-evasive option for treating acne-prone skin. By using avocado as a base you are also providing the skin with a great source of moisturisation that won't leave any excess oil on the skin once cleaned off.

Ingredients:

- ½ of a small ripe avocado, pitted and peeled

- 1 Teaspoon (5ml) Raw organic honey

- ½ Teaspoon (2.5ml) Raw burdock root, finely grated

Instructions:

1. Place the avocado, honey and grated burdock root a mixing bowl and mix well

2. Cleanse your face and neck by means of your usual cleansing routine

3. Apply the avocado, honey and burdock root facial mask to your face and neck, extending down to your décolletage.

4. Leave the mask on for approximately fifteen minutes

5. Gently remove the mask by wiping away at it with a dampened cotton wool pad

6. Follow with your usual cleansing and moisturizing routine.

Pomegranate Juice and Olive Oil Facial Mask

Pomegranates are another super fruit that has become widely known and celebrated for their incredibly high anti-oxidant and anti-aging properties and benefits, so much so that there are many schools of thought who refer to the pomegranate tree as the tree of life. There are a number of commercial cosmetic manufacturers that have begun including pomegranate as an ingredient in their skin care products due to these facts. Olive oil is another super food ingredient that is known in the culinary world for its high content of heart-healthy and cholesterol fighting benefits, however it also has a number of benefits for the skin by both consuming it and applying it topically; olive oil is a wonderful natural moisturizer and will help hydrate the skin without leaving an oily residue. This mask is a wonderful option when looking at fighting the signs of aging.

Ingredients:

- 1 Tablespoon (15ml) Extra virgin olive oil

- 2 teaspoons (10ml) Fresh organic pure pomegranate juice

Instructions:

1. Place the extra virgin olive oil and pomegranate juice into a mixing bowl and mix well

2. Cleanse your face and neck by means of your usual cleansing routine

3. Apply the olive oil and pomegranate juice facial mask to your face and neck, extending down to your décolletage. You may need to use a brush such as a foundation brush or a pastry brush in order to efficiently apply this mask to your skin.

4. Leave the mask on for approximately fifteen minutes

5. Gently remove the mask by wiping away at it with a dampened cotton wool pad

6. Follow with your usual cleansing and moisturizing routine.

Coconut Oil and Melissa Essential Oil Facial Mask

The hyposensitive and calming properties of the Melissa essential oil make it a great addition to any facial product that is intended for use on sensitive skin, or skin that is prone to allergic reactions. Melissa essential oil is also useful in the treatment of acne prone skin or skin that is suffering from some kind of contact dermatitis. The coconut oil provides a gentle, yet effective means of moisturisation and hydration which is something that sensitive skins very often lack, particularly in dry climates.

Ingredients:

- 1 Tablespoon (15ml) Extra virgin organic coconut oil

- ½ Teaspoon (2,5ml) Melissa Essential oil

Instructions:

1. Place the extra virgin coconut oil and Melissa essential oil into a mixing bowl and mix well

2. Cleanse your face and neck by means of your usual cleansing routine

3. Apply coconut oil and Melissa essential oil facial mask to your face and neck, extending down to your décolletage.

4. Leave the mask on for approximately fifteen minutes

5. Gently remove the mask by wiping away at it with a dampened cotton wool pad

6. Follow with your usual cleansing and moisturising routine.

Chapter Three
Homemade Body Scrubs

All the recipes in this section use either Epsom salt or organic sea salt as a base. Epsom salt is a wonderful, cost effective addition to any beauty routine and has so many health benefits due to its high magnesium and sulphate content. Organic sea salt is high in sodium and is one of nature's most simple and effective disinfectants and cleansers. The addition of essential oils to these body scrubs not only adds a hint of gentle fragrance but also brings with it the therapeutic benefits of the essential oils. In some instances food oils such as coconut or olive oil have been added to the mix to boost the moisturising properties of the body scrub. One of the most efficient uses for a body scrub is to exfoliate the skin; exfoliation of the skin removes any excess dead skin cells that may be resting on the skin's surface, paving the way for a more efficient absorption of your moisturising cream. As with all the products and chapters within this book, it is incredibly necessary to stress the fact that if any irritation or sensitivity to the skin is experienced after using any of the following product use of that product must be discontinued immediately, and if any reaction that may be experienced does not clear up within three days of using the product then it is strongly advised that you consult with your doctor or dermatologist.

Epsom Salt and Orange Essential Oil Body Scrub

The high anti-oxidant and anti-aging properties of the orange essential oil, along with the cleansing properties of the Epsom salt make this body scrub a great addition to any beauty routine that takes anti-aging of the entire body into account. Furthermore, the calmative qualities of the orange essential oil fragrance make this a wonderful body scrub to use just before bedtime. Due to the fact that this body scrub is gentle and non-abrasive it is safe to use on the face as well as all over the body.

Ingredients:

- 1 Cup (250ml) Epsom Salt

- 1 Tablespoon (15ml) Orange Essential Oil

Instructions:

1. Place the Epsom salt and the orange essential oil into a mixing bowl that you have set aside for use with non-food items

2. Mix the Epsom salt and the orange essential oil together

3. To use this body scrub on your body take a handful of body scrub and rub over damp skin while in the shower. Make sure that you rinse all the body scrub off of your skin thoroughly before continuing with your usual body cleansing routine.

4. To use the body scrub as a facial exfoliator take a golf ball sized amount of the body scrub and warm it up by rubbing it between

the palms of your hands. Rub the now warmed-up body scrub over your face and neck, extending down to your décolletage. Make sure you have rinsed all the body scrub off of your face thoroughly before continuing with your usual facial cleansing and moisturising routine.

5. This body scrub can be stored in a recycled glass jar and used as and when desired.

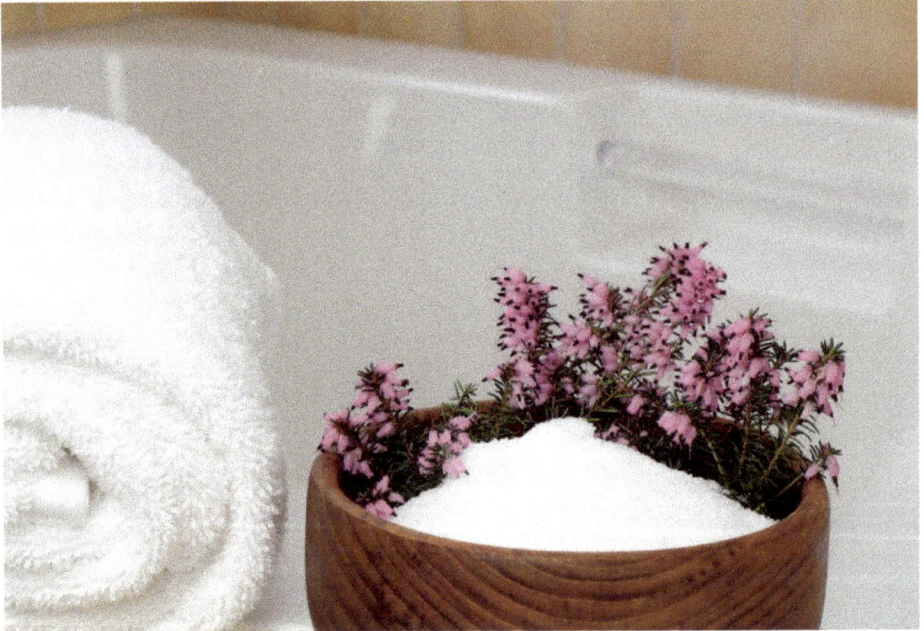

Epsom Salt and Eucalyptus Essential Oil Body Scrub

Eucalyptus essential oil is known for its ability to aid in the release of stiff and sore muscles, therefore when combined with the high magnesium content of the Epsom salt it makes for a wonderful body scrub option after a seriously hard training session. This body scrub can be used in both the shower and the bath, but if you are using it especially for its muscle relaxing properties then it will be best used in conjunction with a long hot soak in the bath. Due to the positive effects that eucalyptus essential oil has on the respiratory system, this body scrub can also be used while recovering from an infection respiratory system; and will also be very helpful as a facial exfoliator in this instance, particularly around the nose and sinus areas of the face.

Ingredients:

- 1 Cup (250ml) Epsom Salt

- 1 Tablespoon (15ml) Eucalyptus essential oil

Instructions:

1. Place the Epsom salt and the eucalyptus essential oil into a mixing bowl that you have set aside for use with non-food items

2. Mix the Epsom salt and the eucalyptus essential oil together

3. To use this body scrub on your body take a handful of body scrub and rub over damp skin while in the shower. Make sure that you

rinse all the body scrub off of your skin thoroughly before continuing with your usual body cleansing routine.

4. To use the body scrub as a facial exfoliator take a golf ball sized amount of the body scrub and warm it up by rubbing it between the palms of your hands. Rub the now warmed-up body scrub over your face and neck, extending down to your décolletage. Make sure you have rinsed all the body scrub off of your face thoroughly before continuing with your usual facial cleansing and moisturising routine.

5. This body scrub can be stored in a recycled glass jar and used as and when desired.

Epsom Salt and Juniper Berry Essential Oil Body Scrub

Juniper berry essential oil is known for its health benefiting properties such as; it is an antiseptic, anti-rheumatic, antispasmodic, calmative, and a diuretic. With its anti-rheumatic properties juniper berry oil will be a great addition to Epsom salt to make a body scrub mixture that will help relieve aching, tired joints and muscles making this body scrub combination another great addition to your after-training soak.

Ingredients:

- 1 Cup (250ml) Epsom Salt

- 1 Tablespoon (15ml) Juniper berry essential oil

Instructions:

1. Place the Epsom salt into a mixing bowl

2. Add the juniper berry essential oil

3. Mix together well, so that all the Epsom salt crystals are well coated with the juniper berry essential oil

4. Place the body scrub mixture into a glass Mason jar and use as desired.

Organic Sea Salt and Coconut Oil Body Scrub

This body scrub both exfoliates and moisturizes the skin at the same time, leaving it feeling soft, supple and ready for the application of any of the homemade moisturizing creams found in chapter one of this book. The vanilla essential oil adds a hint of delicious fragrance to this body scrub, invoking a feeling of comfort and homeliness. Organic sea salt can be quite harsh on the skin so this body scrub is not recommended for very sensitive skins or for use on the face.

Ingredients:

- 1 Cup (250ml) Organic Sea Salt

- ½ Cup (125ml) Extra Virgin Coconut Oil

- 1 Tablespoon (15ml) Vanilla essential oil

Instructions:

1. Place the organic sea salt and the vanilla essential oil into a mixing bowl that you have set aside for use with non-food items

2. Mix in the coconut oil, making sure that all the salt crystals are well covered with the coconut oil and vanilla essential oil

3. To use this body scrub on your body take a handful of body scrub and rub over damp skin while in the shower. Make sure that you rinse all the body scrub off of your skin thoroughly before continuing with your usual body cleansing routine.

4. This body scrub can be stored in a recycled glass jar and used as and when desired.

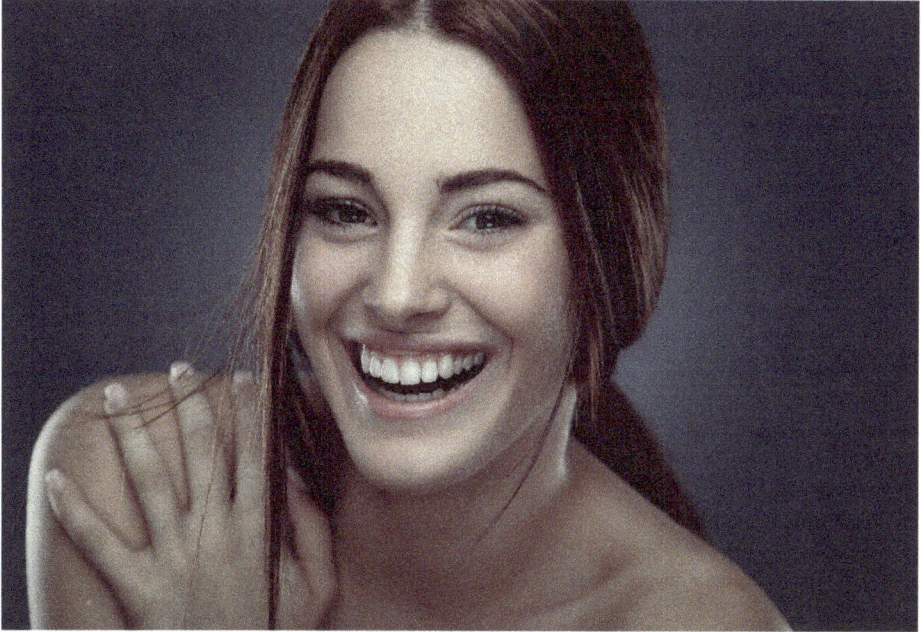

Organic Sea Salt and Olive Oil Body Scrub

This is another body scrub combination that will exfoliate, cleanse and moisturise your skin in one go. The olive oil provides efficient moisturisation and hydration to your skin without leaving it feeling oily and heavy. As with the previous recipe, due to the harshness of the organic sea salt crystals this body scrub is not recommended for use on sensitive skin or as a facial exfoliator.

Ingredients:

- 1 Cup (250ml) Organic Sea Salt

- ½ Cup (125ml) Extra Virgin Olive Oil

Instructions:

1   Place the organic sea salt and the extra virgin olive oil into a mixing bowl

2   Mix in the extra virgin olive oil, making sure that all the salt crystals are well covered with the olive oil

3   To use this body scrub on your body take a handful of body scrub and rub over damp skin while in the shower. Make sure that you rinse all the body scrub off of your skin thoroughly before continuing with your usual body cleansing routine.

4   This body scrub can be stored in a recycled glass jar and used as and when desired

Organic Sea Salt and Avocado Oil Body Scrub

The high potassium and magnesium content of the avocado oil makes this body scrub another great option when looking for an after-training muscle treatment. The motion of rubbing this body scrub over your body before indulging in a long muscle relaxing soak with not only release muscle tension but will exfoliate and moisturise your skin at the same time. As with all the body scrub recipes that use organic sea salt as a base, it is not recommended that this body scrub be used on sensitive skin or as a facial exfoliator.

Ingredients:

- 1 Cup (250ml) Organic Sea Salt

- ½ Cup (125ml) Extra Virgin Avocado Oil

Instructions:

1   Place the organic sea salt and the extra virgin avocado oil into a mixing bowl

2   Mix in the extra virgin avocado oil, making sure that all the salt crystals are well covered with the olive oil

3   To use this body scrub on your body take a handful of body scrub and rub over damp skin while in the shower. Make sure that you

rinse all the body scrub off of your skin thoroughly before continuing with your usual body cleansing routine.

4   This body scrub can be stored in a recycled glass jar and used as and when desired.

Organic Sea Salt, Ginger and Lemongrass Essential Oil Body Scrub

The combination of ingredients in this body scrub makes it a really wonderful option when looking to exfoliate and disinfect the skin at the same time. The anti-inflammatory and anti-bacterial properties of the ginger together with the same properties that are found in the lemongrass essential oil make this body scrub very useful when diluted in warm water as means of cleansing wounds. Once again it is important to note that as with all the organic sea salt based body scrubs found in this book, this body scrub should not be used on sensitive skin nor should it be used as a facial exfoliator.

Ingredients:

- 1 Cup (250ml) Organic Sea Salt

- ½ Cup (125ml) Fresh Ginger root, finely grated

- 1 Tablespoon (15ml) Lemongrass essential oil

Instructions:

1. Place the organic sea salt and finely grated ginger into a mixing bowl

2. Mix in the lemongrass essential oil, making sure that all the salt crystals are well covered with the olive oil and finely grated ginger root

3   To use this body scrub on your body take a handful of body scrub and rub over damp skin while in the shower. Make sure that you rinse all the body scrub off of your skin thoroughly before continuing with your usual body cleansing routine.

4   This body scrub can be stored in a recycled glass jar and used as when desired. It is recommended that this particular body scrub combination be stored in the refrigerator when not in use in order to prevent the fresh ginger root from turning bad.

Organic Sea Salt and Melissa Essential Oil Body Scrub

This body scrub combination is another of those that is very useful when you are looking to ensure complete and thorough cleansing of the skin due to the fact that both ingredients are known for their ability to do so efficiently. Once again it is important to note that since this body scrub is made with an organic sea salt base it is not recommended for use on sensitive skin or as a facial exfoliator.

Ingredients:

- 1 Cup (250ml) Organic Sea Salt

- 1 Tablespoon (15ml) Melissa Essential Oil

Instructions:

1 Place the organic sea salt and Melissa essential oil into a mixing bowl

2 Mix in the Melissa essential oil, making sure that all the salt crystals are well covered with the Melissa essential oil

3 To use this body scrub on your body take a handful of body scrub and rub over damp skin while in the shower. Make sure that you rinse all the body scrub off of your skin thoroughly before continuing with your usual body cleansing routine.

4 This body scrub can be stored in a recycled glass jar and used as when desired.

Chapter Four
Homemade Hair Care Products

Our hair is our crowning glory and taking care of it is an essential part of any beauty routine. The commercial cosmetic industry provides us with a large variety of hair care products that are designed to help strengthen, repair and treat the hair for a number of things from dehydration, damage due to styling and coloring, lack of volume, lack of shine and overall dullness. Unfortunately, as with all products made available by the commercial cosmetic industry, those designed with hair care in mind are also heavily laden with chemical based ingredients that very often can do more harm than good. There is also the factor of price to take into account; many of the commercially available hair care products are very expensive and therefore can become prohibitive and fall into the category of ultimate luxury when on a tight budget. This chapter will give you some creative and interesting ideas for making your own homemade hair care products that will be gentle on your hair and skin as well affordable and cost effective. All the recipes in this chapter use natural ingredients that are easy to source and easy to use. As with all the recipes in previous chapters it is once again very important to stress that should any sensitivity or irritation occur due to use of any of the products in this chapter it is strongly advised that use of the product is discontinued immediately; and that if any reaction that may have occurred does not clear up within three days of using the product then you should consult your doctor or dermatologist.

Coconut Oil Hair Treatment

Pure extra virgin coconut oil makes a wonderful yet simple homemade hair treatment without any serious effort. This recipe has only one ingredient and that is extra virgin coconut oil, which has amazing and very efficient moisturizing properties that are easily absorbed by the hair. Extra virgin coconut oil makes a wonderful, cost effective and easy to use hair treatment for hair that is dry and damaged due to excessive styling and coloring; it is also great to treat hair that is taking strain within hot and dry climates. This treatment will leave your hair feeling hydrated and soft and it is recommended that you use this particular treatment on your hair at least once a month, especially in the case of excessive styling and coloring.

To Use this Treatment:

1   Wash your hair as per your normal shampooing method, but leave out the conditioning step

2   Once you have dried off from your shower, comb out your hair

3   Take a generous amount of coconut oil, preferably in its more solid state, and warm it in between the palms of your hands

4   Work the coconut oil through your hair from root to tip

5   Comb your hair out once again.

6   If you have long hair it will make life easier to braid it and pin it up with hair grips

7   Leave the coconut oil in your hair for twenty four hours before rinsing out and following with your usual shampooing and conditioning routine. You might have to shampoo twice in order to make sure that all the coconut oil has been sufficiently washed out of your hair.

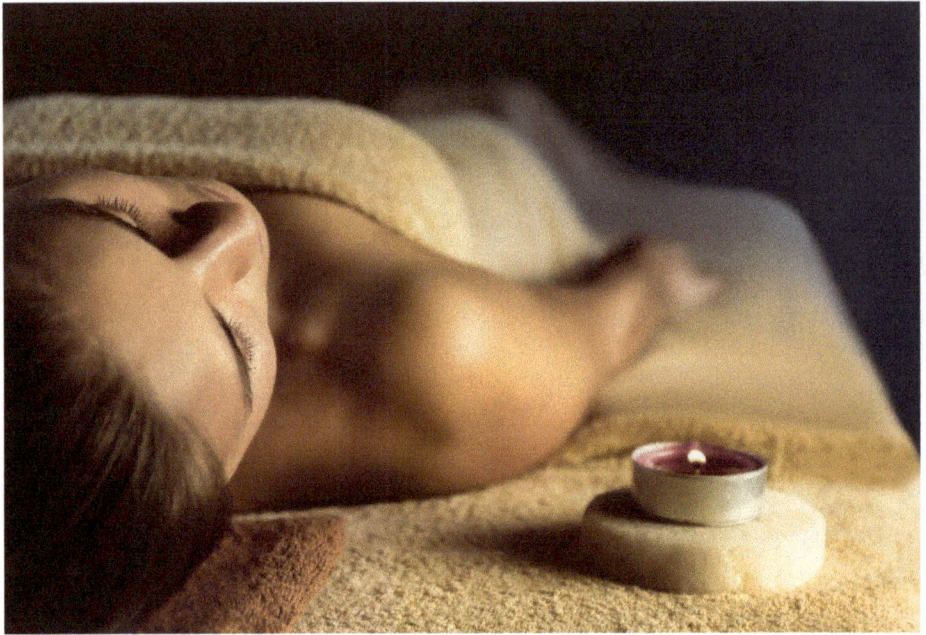

Coconut Oil and Orange Essential Oil Hair Treatment

Due to the amazing properties of orange essential oil such as anti-inflammatory, anti-depressant, anti-spasmodic, it is a natural antiseptic, a carminative, can have a sedative-like effect; it makes a wonderful addition to a homemade hair treatment. The benefits of the orange essential oil can be taken advantage of more efficiently by means of application to the scalp, particularly when we think of the anti-depressant and carminative properties of this particular essential oil. Together with the moisturizing and repairing advantages of the application of pure extra virgin coconut oil has to your hair; the orange essential oil adds a punch of cellular repairing anti-oxidants that are naturally occurring within this essential oil. One of the most pleasant things about this particular hair treatment is the comforting citrus fragrance that is brought on by the addition of the orange essential oil.

Ingredients for this Hair Treatment:

- 1 Cup (250ml) Extra Virgin Coconut oil, preferably in its solid state

- 1 Tablespoon (15ml) Orange essential oil

Instructions to make the hair treatment:

1. In a mixing bowl that you have set aside for use with non-food items, mix together the extra virgin coconut oil and the orange essential oil

2. This hair treatment can be stored in a recycled glass jar and used as and when desired.

To Use this Hair Treatment:

1   Wash your hair as per your normal shampooing method, but leave out the conditioning step

2   Once you have dried off from your shower, comb out your hair

3   Take a generous amount of the coconut oil and orange essential oil hair treatment, preferably in its more solid state, and warm it in between the palms of your hands

4   Work the coconut oil and orange essential oil hair treatment through your hair from root to tip

5   Comb your hair out once again.

6   If you have long hair it will make life easier to braid it and pin it up with hair grips

7   Leave the coconut oil and orange essential oil hair treatment in your hair for twenty four hours before rinsing out and following with your usual shampooing and conditioning routine. You might have to shampoo twice in order to make sure that all the coconut oil has been sufficiently washed out of your hair.

Apple Cider Vinegar Volumizing Hair Treatment

A beautiful shiny and soft main of hair that is full of body and bounce is something that is sure to put a spring in our step should we be able to achieve such a thing on any given day. Many of the products made available to us by the cosmetic industry are chemical-based and highly fragranced, which can lead to irritations for people with sensitive skin. Also the extended use of styling products can lead to a build-up of these products in our hair causing it to be weighed down and look dull and lifeless.

Apple cider vinegar contains a high acetic acid content and is a natural alternative to the products made available by the cosmetic industry for such concern. The use of apple cider vinegar on your hair will naturally remove the build-up of styling products and at the same time strengthen the hair shaft, resulting in a healthy hair follicle that will in turn produce and grow a healthier, shinier strand of hair. Apple cider vinegar will also help to restore the natural pH balance of the scalp and hair shafts resulting in an increase in hair growth and volume.

Ingredients for this hair treatment:

- ¼ Cup (60ml) Organic apple cider vinegar

- 4 Cups (1litre) Pure spring water, at a lukewarm temperature

Instructions:

1   In a large jug, mix the organic apple cider vinegar with the pure spring water

2   Transfer the apple cider vinegar and water solution into a spray bottle.

To use this hair treatment:

1   Wash your hair as per your normal shampooing method, but leave out the conditioning step

2   Once you have dried off from your shower, comb out your hair

3   Spray the apple cider vinegar generously over your damp hair, making sure that you apply a good amount of the solution to your scalp working down the hair shaft

4   Allow this solution to sit in your hair for approximately five minutes before rinsing off thoroughly with cold water. It is necessary to use cold water to rinse this solution off your hair is the cold temperature will help seal the hair shaft resulting in the shine and bounce that you are wanting to achieve for your hair by using this particular treatment.

Olive Oil and Lavender Essential Oil Hair Treatment

Due to the fact that lavender essential oil is known for its ability to relieve and eliminate nervous tension, relieve pain, disinfect the skin and enhance respiratory function. The addition of lavender essential oil to this hair treatment further helps your body reap these amazing benefits of this essential oil simply because you are applying it to your scalp and since our heads are generally the primary source of generation for nervous tension, it just makes sense to add lavender essential oil to a hair treatment. The extra virgin olive oil will provide your hair and scalp with intense moisturisation and will also help to repair your locks from any damage that has been done due to excessive styling and coloring of the hair.

Ingredients to make this hair treatment:

- 1 Cup (250ml) Extra Virgin Olive Oil

- 1 Tablespoon (15ml) Lavender essential oil

Instructions to make this hair treatment:

1   Mix the extra virgin olive oil together with the lavender essential oil in a jug that you have set aside for use with non-food items.

2   Pour the olive and lavender essential oil mixture into a small recycled glass jar

3   This hair treatment can be used as and when desired

To Use this Hair Treatment:

1   Wash your hair as per your normal shampooing method, but leave out the conditioning step

2   Once you have dried off from your shower, comb out your hair

3   Take a generous amount of the olive oil and lavender essential oil hair treatment, and warm it in between the palms of your hands

4   Work the olive oil and lavender essential oil hair treatment through your hair from root to tip, making sure that you take the time to massage it into your scalp so that the hair cuticles can reap benefit from the ingredients in this hair treatment.

5   Comb your hair out once again.

6   If you have long hair it will make life easier to braid it and pin it up with hair grips

7   Leave the olive oil and lavender essential oil hair treatment in your hair for twenty four hours before rinsing out and following with your usual shampooing and conditioning routine. You might have to shampoo twice in order to make sure that all the olive oil and lavender essential oil has been sufficiently washed out of your hair.

Conclusion

The overall aim of this book was to illustrate in as clear a way as possible how easy it is to achieve a balance in your beauty and body care routine that does not wholly rely on the commercially manufactured cosmetics that are made available to us on our supermarket and drug store shelves. This book further sought to provide healthy, non-abrasive, affordable and easily obtainable beauty care products for those who suffer from sensitive skin and are prone to developing allergies to the vast amounts of chemicals that commercially manufactured cosmetic products are made up of. Since all the ingredients that are used in the making of these homemade beauty products are natural products they do not promote the cruelty to animals and the testing of products on animals in any way at all, allowing you to use all of these products with a completely clear conscious and peace of mind that you are in no way causing harm to nature or the environment.

As a last note, it is once again very necessary to remind you that all of the products and recipes in this book should be used with absolute caution and that if any irritation or sensitivity is experienced due to the use of any of these products it is very strongly advised that you discontinue use of the product immediately. Furthermore if any reaction to any of the products or recipes in this book does not clear up within three days of the discontinuation of use of the product, it is strongly advised that you consult with your doctor or dermatologist.

Finally, if you have a second, please review this book.

Even one sentence review will do and I'd be really happy to hear from you!

I hope you will enjoy your holistic health and beauty journey!

I hope to "see" you in my next book.

Wishing you all the best,

Cassia

You Will Find More Books at:

www.YourWellnessBooks.com

www.LOAforSuccess.com

Notes:

www.ingramcontent.com/pod-product-compliance
Lightning Source LLC
Chambersburg PA
CBHW041217030426
42336CB00023B/3378